How to Quit Drinking

How to Quit Drinking

End the brain fog, improve your mental sharpness, escape the cultural hypnosis, and have more energy. Why life is better without booze.

By Karl Whitfield

The one-hour wisdom series.
Small Books: Big Ideas

How to Quit Drinking - End the brain fog, improve your mental sharpness, escape the cultural hypnosis, and have more energy. Why life is better without booze.
By Karl Whitfield

Book one in the One-Hour Wisdom series. Small Books: Big Ideas

ISBN 9798620577132

Karl Whitfield has asserted his right under the Copyright, Designs and Patents Act 1988 to be identified as the author of this work.

This book is a work of non-fiction based on the life, experiences and recollections of the author. Please refer to the medial disclaimer in the end papers. All product and company names are trademarks of their respective owners. Neither Karl Whitfield nor MND Health Ltd has any affiliation or commercial relationship with any companies or products named within this document.

All rights reserved. This document is protected under copyright. No part of this publication may not be copied other than for non-commercial individual reference with all copyright or other proprietary notices retained, and thereafter may not be recopied, reproduced, displayed in the public domain or otherwise redistributed without the express written permission of the publisher.

Cover design by Fizart Design.

© Karl Whitfield. Copyright 2020

Contents

Beginning 1
You Booze, You Lose 3
My Own Story 7
30 Days to Eight Years 11
The Health Burden 15
Your Challenge 21
Your First Year 25
The Best Version of You 29
To Your Future 31
One-Hour Wisdom 33
More 35
Legal Disclaimer 37

Beginning

This is not a book about alcoholism. This book is probably not going to be a huge help to alcoholics. I am not an alcoholic, I was never an alcoholic, and I am not qualified nor experienced enough to offer dependent drinkers the professional help they need.

This is a book about drinking alcohol. This book is for the many millions who are not dependent alcoholics, but drink more than they should, and perhaps are not fully aware of the harm it's doing to their health, their mental wellbeing, and society at large.

This book is for all those people who like a drink or two every day, or most days, who don't fully realise they are drinking too much. It's a book about the social hypnosis and cultural normalisation of drinking, and how it poisons your body and clouds your mind.

I believe that for most of us, life without booze, is better.

How to Quit Drinking

You Booze, You Lose

Drinking sucks. In my opinion there are millions of people out there who drink more than they really should, and they are blind to the harm that it causes. This is not a book about alcoholism.

Alcoholism is a disease, not a choice. One of the defining factors of alcoholism is that it affects the way your brain works. It affects your ability to think rationally. Once alcohol takes a grip in your brain, you think about drinking all the time, you feel cravings for drink, you no longer function completely normally and you can't make rational, intelligent decisions about your own drinking.

Alcoholism, like some other addictions, stops your brain from working completely normally.

You have a choice

No one chooses to become an alcoholic. But *maybe we can choose* to see the descent into alcoholism as a continuum, a progression, like a descending staircase.

We can stand on the **top step**, totally sober, a teetotaller, and we can choose, freely, whether to have 'one drink per month' or 'one drink per week' or 'one drink per day' or 'several drinks every day'.

Perhaps, one drink per *month* is the **first step** down the staircase.

Perhaps, one drink per *week* is the **second step**.

If we buy this analogy, then maybe one drink per *day* is the **third step**. Still, no big deal, there are many millions of people who drink that much, a glass of wine over dinner every evening, a beer from the fridge when you get home from work. An average of seven drinks per week. Some weeks it's five drinks, some weeks it's 10, but it's an average of seven. That's 'one drink per day'.

Down to the next step, the **fourth step**. Now it's two drinks per day, two glasses of wine or two beers, on average, every day. Again, millions of people do that. An average of 14 drinks per week. I was doing that, sometimes a little less, sometimes (often) a fair bit more, for many years.

The **fifth step**. Several drinks per day. Two to five, an average of 20 to 30 drinks per week. Again, there are plenty doing that, millions of people.

And now we descend...the **sixth step**, the **seventh step**, the **eighth step**...now we are into the realm of 'drunk nearly every day' and we start to see people suffering some of the immediate, visible health problems associated with drinking. Now we are into alcoholism, addiction, dependency.

Alcoholism is a disease. It affects normal brain function. No one would knowingly, purposefully *choose* to become an alcoholic.

But at one point in time, we all stand on that top step. And we can choose...to stay on the top step, or go down to the first step, or the second step, or the third, or the fourth.

We may have lost control by the seventh step. Stepping from seventh to eighth, from eighth to ninth, these may be symptoms of the disease, rather than free choices, but stepping from the first step to the second, *is free choice*. From the second step to the third, **is** *rational choice*, a decision you **can** control.

I believe millions of people live on the second, third, fourth and fifth step, perhaps drinking something between two drinks per week and three drinks per day.

This is choice, not alcoholism, but free choice.
This book, is for those people.

I believe that drinking every day, or almost every day, five to seven days per week, one, two or three drinks per day, averaging around 15 to 20 drinks per week, is harmful to our health in ways that most people fail to understand. Personally, I was in that zone for 26 years.

It's not alcoholism, but in my opinion it's the beginnings of dependency, it's a disordered habit that many find extremely hard to break. I speak to a lot of people who drink that amount, and say they have no dependency, they are not addicted, they just enjoy it.

They say they are not addicted, until they try to go a week without a drink.

If one of the symptoms of alcoholism is that you think about drinking a lot, you crave drink, and you lack the ability to make rational decisions around your drinking, then it seems to me that the descent into mental illness exists on a scale.

You could choose to see it like this, if you wanted to:

- Drinking one drink per week, step two on our 'staircase analogy', no problem at all.
- Drinking eight or nine drinks per day, step seven on our staircase, dependency problem.

Maybe there is a line between those two points. And if there is such a line, I would guess that the point where we cross from 'controllable social habit' to 'dependent and can't stop' *differs for each of us* - likely depending on our physical body size, genetic predispositions, mental wellbeing, age, certain metabolic factors, other dietary and lifestyle habits, our social environment, and more. While one person may become a dependent drinker at only three or four units per day, another person may not cross that line until they are drinking two or three times that much.

Insidious poison

My wise and kind friend describes alcohol as 'an insidious poison'. The definition of 'insidious' is: proceeding in a gradual, subtle way, but with very harmful effects.

This perfectly describes alcohol.

Drinking is such a material part of our culture, it's seen as the norm, indeed teetotallers are seen as the odd ones out. When we quit drinking and tell our friends, we face comments like *"Really, why, what's wrong with you?"* and *"Why would you do that, how boring!"* Many people fear *"If I quit, my friends will think I'm boring."*

Marketers sell alcohol to us with imagery that suggests drinking is what the cool people do, it's what the beautiful, sexy people do, it's all fun and laughter. But reality isn't like that. Sure, moderate drinking can be fun, but moderate drinking all-too-often leads to heavy drinking.

Drinking often breeds violence. Street violence, domestic violence, child abuse. There is nothing funny about puddles of vomit on our pavements. There is nothing sexy about passing out and pissing yourself.

When I quit, some friends were amazed *"You've stopped drinking?!?!? Oh, how boring!"* they would blurt out, mouth spouting before the brain had a chance to think it through.

I learned to quickly retort, with a deadpan expression, *"Are you saying I'm boring when I'm sober?"*

I would hold my serious face for a few seconds, as awkward embarrassment ensued...then I'd fall into laughter *"Ahaha, got you, ha ha you didn't know what to say!!"* and it would all be fun, and my friends would know I was just teasing them. But the underlying thought is real, and is serious. We hold a societal notion that drinking is cool, fun, aspirational, and that teetotal is boring, as if to suggest that being sober is to somehow miss out on all the fun.

Don't buy into that cultural bullshit. It's a lie, and it's doing you harm.

Drinking sucks

In my opinion, it steals from you, slowly drains your energy, it takes the best of you. I think the descent from 'a couple of drinks per week' which is pretty harmless, innocuous and may even be beneficial to your health as a stress reliever, down to alcoholic dependency, occurs as a series of steps, a slippery slope.

Don't play the victim. While people on the lower half of that staircase have become *casualties of the disease of alcohol*, people on the top are in **full control**. That's who this book is aimed at, and those people still have freedom of choice.

I believe that drinking clouds your mind, it's a social hypnosis, an insidious poison, you don't see it getting a grip on you, but believe me, it does. For the overwhelming majority of us, we're better off without it.

You booze, you lose.

My Own Story

My own story around alcohol is nothing remarkable. Maybe, however, that's exactly the point. I was just doing what millions of other people do. I wasn't an alcoholic, but I was drinking enough to have a negative impact on my health, to contribute to my obesity, to cloud my mind and render me weary, always wanting another couple of hours in bed in the morning.

Other people have probably written books about overcoming their alcohol addiction, and they probably have remarkable stories to tell, of the shocking or humiliating things they have done under the influence. Well this isn't a book about overcoming addiction; this is more a book about not falling into addiction in the first place; a book about recognising the slippery slope, and turning yourself around before things go too far.

Shitfaced

Don't get me wrong, I did my share of getting shitfaced. As a teen, and in my twenties, I spent years partying as hard as anyone. Over 15 years, I embarrassed myself plenty of times with my outrageous behaviour.

I was a fairly wayward youth. I would smoke three packs a day, drink until I vomit several nights per week, and experiment with all manner of other substances. But for all the drugs we tried, I was old school, I always came back to booze. Beer and whisky were my drugs of choice, they were dependable, like old friends.

Certainly, as a youth, I was a very heavy drinker, and there were plenty of times it brought out the worst in me. Especially whisky, which made me an extremely unfriendly 250-pound (113 kg) monster. Of course, there were 'funny' stories, hilarious escapades that ended in being escorted home by police officers, antics dancing around naked in the snow, long nights that involved drinking through until daybreak. And there were less attractive stories too, things I am certainly not proud of. Vandalism, cars wrecked, and street fights that didn't end well, my face bruised and bleeding.

But I don't look back on those times as problematic. I was a typical 'angry young man' and booze was just an outlet. I drank heavily in those days, but it seemed normal; everyone around me drank too, I was just exceedingly proficient at it.

Adult life

The years that I have an issue with, were after my misspent youth. As an adult, a husband and father, with a responsible job, a role model for my children.
And this isn't a story about the *quantity* I would drink.
It's a story about my poor *relationship* with drink.
Over the decade from my mid-twenties to my mid-thirties, I had grown up to be a 'sensible family man'. I got married, we had kids, I had a house, a mortgage, bills to pay. I got a decent job, then in my thirties I set up and ran my own business; I had staff, taxes to pay, deadlines to meet. I was a grown up now, I had responsibilities.
But when I thought about alcohol, I was struck by three things.

One: I could be a real arsehole sometimes. I said some mean things to people I care about. It might be an argument with my girlfriend, or later with my wife, a disagreement with a friend, or an exchange with a stranger, but if alcohol was inside me, I could be harsh, judgemental, quick to anger, and slow to apologise. I think alcohol brings out the worst in a lot of people. Not for everyone, and not always, but often. It did in me, certainly beer and spirits, less so wine.

Two: I was living with a low level but permanent version of what many people call 'brain fog' but I didn't really know it at the time. Personally, I think a lot of people live this way. We might blame it on stress, tiredness, the weather, the economy, or myriad other things; it's just there, a subtle but pervading sense of overwhelm, that everything is a bit too much, like we're permanently playing catch-up, just trying to make sense of everything, but never quite coming out on top.

Three: I didn't have a healthy relationship with alcohol. In truth, this is the big one, the main reason I stopped drinking. I liked to drink every day, and as each year passed, I found this habit ever-more present. I found I was opening a bottle of wine over dinner every night, two on a

Friday, two on a Saturday, sometimes more depending who I was with, plus a few beers on a Saturday and Sunday afternoon. Sharing with my wife, we were getting through ten bottles of wine each week, often more, and I was always drinking the bigger half of each bottle, and I didn't want to take a night off.

This bothered me, but I didn't realise it bothered me, I didn't acknowledge that thought in the back of my mind, until a good friend posed this simple question to me…

> *"How would it make you feel if you were to go 30 days without a drink?"*

I thought about the question for a short while, and then I answered honestly, *"I'd be terrified! Bloody hell, to get to 6pm on a Friday evening, or 'wine o'clock' as I like to call it, after a hard week at work, and not open a bottle of red wine, would be unbearable."*

My friend asked me to take a moment, to reconsider my answer, to be sure I meant it, sure I was serious, and then to reflect on how that made me feel.

I contemplated, and my answer was yes, I was dead serious. Frankly, the thought of going a weekend without a drink terrified me, let alone going a whole month. I felt I could abstain on a week night, in fact I sometimes did, we would sometimes pick a random Tuesday or Thursday and decide to have a night off alcohol, because it seemed like a sensible, healthy thing to do from time to time, but I felt there was absolutely no way I could go through a Friday night or Saturday night without a drink! Torture!

Answering his questions, I realised…

> *Alcohol had more of a hold on me than I had previously acknowledged. Alcohol was perhaps in control of me, somewhat more than I was in control of it.*

And that really pissed me off.

Because I like to think I am in control of my life. I like to think I'm some kind of tough guy, and smart, and I've got my shit together.

It annoyed me to realise that something as silly as a few mouthfuls of some innocuous looking red liquid swilling around in a glass, could have such a powerful influence on my life.

My challenge

My friend and I discussed my feelings, and he challenged me, gently, without pushing, to consider trying it; 30 days without a drink.

No pressure. Just give it a try.

I did. Not that day, to be honest, I spent a few days thinking about it and mentally preparing for it, but then I went 30 days without a drink.

I found the first week or so very hard, very awkward, it felt weird. Breaking an established habit can be hard. But once I had done a week, particularly a weekend, then it eased, as my brain told me 'if you can do one week, you can do another!'

I got through the 30 days, and it hadn't been as hard as I feared, and I felt a certain sense of pride in my accomplishment. After the 30 days, I immediately started drinking again. But that challenge had sown a seed. Deep in my mind, a thought was now germinating 'Fuck you alcohol, I can be in control, I can show you who's boss.'

30 Days to Eight Years

Over time, as this seed germinated, I began to think I could try a harder challenge. The 30-day challenge had been a success, and actually, after the first 10 days, it hadn't really been too hard. I got through those first 10 days on sheer will power, I'm a determined kinda guy so will power is something I'm pretty good at, then after that, it wasn't too bad.

But what if I tried a longer challenge? I told myself that 30 days is not long, but if I tried something longer, additional hurdles are going to crop up.

I fancied trying 90 days. That seemed like the next logical step after 30 days. But at that time in my life, in my late thirties, a family man, business owner, a gregarious outgoing sort of chap with lots of friends, any period of 90 days is likely to include a wedding or a big birthday party, a family holiday, Christmas party, or some other such major event that would involve drinking.

Surviving 30 days mostly at home without a drink was one thing, but how would I survive a major social function completely sober?

Designated driver

My wife always enjoyed drinking wine with me, but she never drank as much as me. When we drank at home, I always drank the lion's share. When we went out, she would generally drive more often than me.

I figured I could be designated driver. This would be my excuse. When folks offered me a drink and I said no, it would be a potential minefield to say *"No, thanks, I'm not drinking alcohol at the moment."* Good grief, there would be too many questions, weird looks, it just wouldn't fly.

But if I said *"Not for me thanks, I'm driving"* that would fly. I noticed when my wife said she was driving, no one gave her any crap about that, they generally just said *"Oh bad luck!"* or something like that, without questioning her motives, because we all understand driving.

90 days

With my designated driver excuse tucked up my sleeve, I tackled 90 days. Again, it was the first week or two I found hardest, but I knew I had done it before, so mentally the challenge was much easier the second time around. I think, for me, the second challenge was totally different, my mental approach was totally different.

I mean, the first time, doing the 30-day challenge, it was something I didn't really want to do. I didn't really want to abstain from drinking, I bloody love wine, I love the taste, and I absolutely love drinking the stuff! But I did it because I *wanted* to test myself, to *beat the challenge*, and prove I could be in control, just a tiny bit more than I wanted to drink another 30 days' worth of delicious red wine!

But the second challenge, for 90 days, was different. Now, this test was something I set for myself, it wasn't a challenge from my friend, it was self-set. Now we had the version of me that wants to drink delicious wine every day, up against the version of me who loves a challenge and loves to win!

Damn! I'm a pretty competitive guy, so I think this time I was far more motivated to make it work, because I love testing myself, in sports, in business, in life. I think the 90 days was easier than the original 30 days, for this reason, because mentally, I *wanted* to complete the challenge. **I wanted to win.**

And I did.

And after 90 days, I definitely felt health benefits for my abstinence. I had lost weight, I was less tired, and I felt more spring in my step.

Tastes bitter as hell

Oddly, on day 91, I couldn't wait to chug down a nice cold beer! It was summer time, a warm sunny day, and having completed my challenge the day before, I couldn't wait to get my hands on the ice-cold beers I had chilling in my fridge ready for me.

The first one tasted like shit!

Now this was quite a revelation to me. The first beer tasted bitter as hell. I gulped it down in minutes, but it tasted pretty awful. I remember thinking *'Wow, this is an acquired taste, how the heck did I ever grow to like these things in the first place?'*

I decided the only way to cure this odd taste was to have another, and by the time I had finished the second bottle, I was 'cured' and loving the taste again!

I think there's a lesson in there somewhere!!

The big one: One Year!

Some time passed, maybe another 18 months, and at first, after my 90-day experiment, for a few months I definitely drank a little less. I think some more seeds had been planted in my mind, and those ideas were taking time to grow.

As the months went by, the drinking became heavier again, and in fact even more so than before, and it started draining my energy again. I was on a real personal health transformation, I had lost a ton of weight, quit smoking, I was feeling lighter and fitter than I had at any time in the previous 20 years, but somehow that made the booze more of a burden.

As a hard drinker I had always been strong as an ox when it came to shaking off any kind of hangover. I was that guy, back in my twenties, who could get wasted, puke, then have just three- or four-hours sleep, grab a strong coffee and be ready for action at 7am the next morning.

But here I was aged 40, and now two bottles of red wine on Friday night, would leave me feeling jaded and below-par all weekend. I didn't like that. It seemed to run counter to every other effort I was making to embrace healthy living. *It didn't feel like who I wanted to be any more.*

Let's just run that last line again.

It didn't feel like who I wanted to be any more.

(**Hint:** magic secret right there. I changed my identity, inside, I changed who I was. I now identified myself as a healthy person, and suddenly, getting blitzed and then feeling like shit afterwards, didn't really float my boat anymore!)

As time went on, in my mind, I started cooking up the mother of all challenges. **One year without a drink.**

New Year's Eve was only a few weeks away. It seemed the obvious opportunity, could I do a full calendar year.

We used to host a New Year's party in our house every year. We had young kids at primary school, and lots of our friends did too. No one can ever get a baby sitter on New Year's Eve, so to make life easy, we used to have everyone to us - a dozen or so adults, and a dozen or so young kids. It was always lots of fun.

I figured I would toast in the New Year with our friends, finish my drink by a few minutes after midnight, then not drink again until the New Year's toast the following year.

And that's exactly what I did. We threw a party, had a great night, I drank lots throughout the evening, toasted in the New Year at midnight, put my glass down empty within the next 15 minutes, and then did not drink for a year.

Best. Thing. Ever.

At the end of one year, I felt so good, and I felt I had benefitted so much from become a teetotaller, that staying sober was a no-brainer. You'd have had to pay me, a lot, to start drinking again.

It's had a massive and profound effect on my health, and my life. My brain has never worked so well, my thinking never been so clear.

When the full year rolled around, the following New Year's Eve party I stayed sober, I vowed to keep going and I haven't had a drink since. As this book is going to print, it's now been eight years and two months since I had a drink, and I'm still loving the feeling.

The health benefits have been profound.

The mental benefits have been profound.

Along the way, I'm sure I must have saved a small fortune in cash terms! (Beer mat calculations: 8 years is 400 weeks, 60 quid per week = 25 grand saved!)

As my kids are now all teenagers, I'm glad they have no recollection of ever seeing me drunk; my gut feel says that makes me a better parental influence on them.

The Health Burden

Alcohol has a lot of known negative health consequences. The cost to society is massive. According to the World Health Organization (WHO), drinking contributes to a staggering 200 different health conditions, including obesity, sexual dysfunction, liver disease, breast and bowel cancer, depression, behavioural disorders and degenerative neurological conditions.

The WHO states that alcohol causes 5.3% of all deaths worldwide annually, amounting to over three million people.

According to the Centres for Disease Control and Prevention (CDC), excessive drinking kills over 88,000 people in the United States every year.

According to Cancer Research UK, 4% of all cancer in the UK is directly attributable to drinking alcohol, making it the fourth leading preventable cause of cancer in the UK. Drinking alcohol contributes to seven types of cancer, including breast cancer, and can lead to liver damage and liver disease.

According to the American Cancer Society, "Alcohol use has been linked with cancers of the mouth, throat, larynx, oesophagus, liver, colon, rectum, and breast. Alcohol may also increase the risk of cancers of the pancreas and stomach. For each of these cancers, the more alcohol you drink, the higher your cancer risk."

Read that last line again. "The more alcohol you drink, the higher your cancer risk."

Remember, **you have a choice.**

Yet, a lot of people don't know this. Cancer Research UK found in a survey that 87% of the British public were not particularly aware that drinking contributed to cancer.

When asked what ill health was caused by drinking, only 13% mentioned cancer.

Financial costs

The cost to our society is massive. In the US, the CDC states that *"The cost of excessive alcohol use in the United States reached $249 billion in 2010. Most (77%) of these costs were due to binge drinking. Binge drinking is defined as drinking four or more alcoholic beverages per occasion for women or five or more drinks per occasion for men."*

In the UK, the Institute of Alcohol Studies *"estimates that the total social cost of alcohol to England in 2006-07 was £55.1 billion"* and Public Health England states that *"Alcohol is now more affordable and people are drinking more than they did in the past. Between 1980 and 2008, there was a 42% increase in the sale of alcohol."* And *"The economic burden of health, social and economic alcohol-related harm is substantial, with estimates placing the annual cost to be between 1.3% and 2.7% of annual GDP."*

It's a poison

When we read those facts, the stark reality of how harmful alcohol is becomes quite undeniable. Alcohol is costing society so much, in health care costs, social disorder and lost productivity, that it is actually negating GDP growth. Seriously, UK GDP growth from the post-crash period 2009, to 2019, was only around 1.5% average. The societal cost of alcohol wipes out more than that every year. We are retarding our own economic growth as a nation because we are addicted to drinking too much. That's just crazy.

Alcohol consumption is killing over three million people every year, and contributing to a wide range of physical and mental health problems, and yet it is widely and easily available, and actively, legally, marketed…particularly to young adults!

Think about that! It makes no sense…

> *"Hey there, bright young minds, you are the future of our nation, here, get fucked up on this stuff! It will rot your brain, give you cancer and you'll die young, but ha ha, who cares, because it tastes nice, and it's cool and sexy!"*

Utter madness.
Seriously, alcohol is a poison. People need to understand this.

If I invented a new product, today, a liquid that you can consume...

- One small glassful, and you'll feel slightly relaxed, and laugh more.
- Two glasses and you might feel more confident, talkative, a little louder than usual.
- Three glasses and you shouldn't drive or operate machinery, your judgement and coordination might be impaired.
- Four glasses you might fall over, bump into things and other people, slur your words, become aggressive, get into a fight.
- Five glasses you might vomit, and you'll probably say mean things to people you love, call them names and start an argument.
- Six glasses and it's likely you'll be sick, pass out, break stuff, fall down stairs.
- Seven glasses and you're certain to be ill and throw up and fall asleep in a puddle of your own sick. You could easily fall off a bridge, walk in front of a vehicle or get yourself arrested.
- Eight glasses and you might have a mild form of blood poisoning and need to go to hospital for a stomach pump!
- Oh, and by the way, regular use of this stuff causes addiction, brain fog, obesity, erectile dysfunction, depression, liver disease, stomach cancer and lots more.

If I invented this today as a new product, and went to seek approval to sell this substance to the public, coloured to make it look nice, flavoured with some fruit juice, packaged in a cool attractive bottle, and I intend to get very rich marketing it to impressionable young people...**I would be laughed out of the room!**

No *sane* food and drug approval board in any country in the world would allow such a poison to be legally sold to the public, and yet, that's what we have with alcohol.

Worse than smoking

Given the facts laid out above, the health harms, the damage to mental wellbeing, the societal cost, and the many millions living with 'brain fog' not even realising that their two-drinks-per-day beer or wine habit is the cause, personally, I'd sooner start smoking again than drinking, I think it's that harmful.

No exaggeration.

In fact, in my live seminars I often ask my audience to consider this hypothetical scenario.

If I came to you on, say, your 20th birthday, and gave you a pack of 20 cigarettes, and I said *"smoke these today, I'll give you another pack tomorrow"* and then I gave you a pack every day until your 50th birthday, what harm might that do your health?

I have posed this question many times, and I find audiences will shout out *"lung cancer"* and *"bronchitis"* and *"emphysema"* and more. There is a long list of possible health problems you might suffer from smoking a pack-a-day for 30 years.

But then I ask, what if instead of giving you 20 cigarettes, I gave you 20 chocolate-chip cookies? And you ate them all, and then I gave you 20 more the next day, and every day for 30 years. What might that do to your health?

My audiences will call out *"obesity", "diabetes", "high blood pressure", "heart disease"* and much more besides.

Then I ask, what if it was 20 alcoholic drinks? 20 shots, or 20 glasses of wine, or 20 bottles of beer? If I gave you 20 drinks every day, what would that do to your health over 30 years?

At this point, audiences often fall silent and look dumbstruck, contemplating something they have never considered before, until someone usually calls out *"You'd probably be dead."*

I've done this in live events for years, and my audiences generally conclude that the drinking scenario would be the most harmful. I once had a doctor in the room who stood up and said *"Of those three, without a doubt, the drinking would do the most harm, then the sugar, and the smoking probably the least."* I am inclined to agree with him.

The key point is to understand is that we need to view drinking alcohol the way we view smoking. It's harmful, it kills. A little, in moderation, is sustainable, but frequent and regular use for a long time, kills.

Know the risks

As stated previously, Cancer Research UK found that only 13% of the British population understand that drinking is a causal factor in several common cancers, including breast cancer, the most prevalent cancer in females in both the UK and the United States.

87% of people did not know.

Well, now, *you* do know.

Now, you have the information. You can now change your habits, to help yourself, to reduce your risk.

You have a choice.

How to Quit Drinking

Your Challenge

Over the first four chapters you have read about the harm alcohol is doing to your health, about the harm it does to our society, and about how it drains you of energy, clouds your mind and depresses brain function. You've also read about my own journey, and how I started with a simple challenge - don't drink for 30 days.

Now, in this chapter, it's over to you.

Your turn.

Your challenge.

This isn't *me* setting you a challenge. I don't know you, and I don't know what day, month, or year you are reading this book. I can't set you the challenge, but *you* can.

This is your decision, your test, your challenge. You need to do this - for you. Not because some guy who wrote a book challenged you, but for yourself, because you believe in yourself, because you have proactively chosen to participate in your own destiny. Because you know what's right, and you want to be the best version of you that you can possibly be.

30 days

> *Can you go for 30 days, just one month of your adult life, without drinking any alcohol?*

Personally, I don't think this is about willpower, I don't think this is about mind over matter. Willpower is great and all that, there are times it's a very useful and powerful force, and it's going to help you in those first few days, but for the full 30 days, I don't think it's the be-all, end-all solution.

What worked for me was a change of mindset. It was two-fold.

Firstly, I *wanted to prove to myself* that I can be in control, that I was strong, that I wasn't prepared to let this silly little glass of liquid have so much power over me, I was 'better' than that. (These are my personal feelings, I'm not projecting them on to you, just sharing them with you. I'm not suggesting that sober people are 'better' than people who drink, or that people who drink are 'weak people'. I'm just sharing the *internal dialogue from my own mind*. For me, being under the control of this drug made *me* feel 'weak', and taking back control made *me* feel 'better', like I was accomplishing some great personal victory. That was **my internal language**. What's yours?)

Secondly, I changed my *internal self-identity*. At this time, for me, addressing my relationship with alcohol was the next really major hurdle in a broader life transformation. It was part of my quest to 'become a healthy person'. I lost 101 pounds of fat (46 kilos), quit smoking after 20 years, got fit, started running marathons and lifting weights, qualified as a Personal Trainer and started building some muscle. Tackling my drinking was a part of that transformation in my life.

I don't think I ever set out to become teetotal. I just wanted to get back in control. I think I would have liked to become a 'sociable drinker' like some people do so well. Some weeks include just two or three drinks. Some weeks include a half-a-dozen or more. Some weeks, none. I quietly admire people who have that healthy, controlled relationship with alcohol. But I could never do that, such was my relationship with alcohol that I was all, or nothing.

All or nothing

That's probably an important factor in all this. 'All or nothing' is very much the kind of person I am. I am that guy in business, in sports, in relationships, in personal endeavours, tests, challenges, studying, learning a new skill, anything! I'm all in, or all out, there is no half way.

Personally, I find total abstinence easier than pacing myself.

I know there are lots of books, systems and methods out there to help people drink less. I never found such systems work for me - not with smoking, drinking, eating or any other habit change. There are these systems of 'only xx many units per week' or 'only drink on two days in each week' or 'adding up the drinks, or allocating points' or 'only drink on special occasions' but personally I don't get on with such systems. **You might**, but I didn't.

I tried all those things and they never worked for me. It's too stressful trying to remember what day it is and what you are supposed to do. It means you are always thinking about drinking.

As a health and weight loss coach, I have coached a number of people to quit drinking, and almost invariably, by the time they come to work with me, they have tried a few of those systems before on their own.

I ask those people to tell me what they have tried so far, and then I just listen to the stories. I hear the confusion and complexity. *"Well I was supposed to only be drinking two days in any week, but then we had to attend Uncle Mick's 50th birthday bash and then I was at my friend's wedding, and that week I drank three times, so I though the next week I would only drink once, but then I had a hell of a week at work, so I had a few, and then..."*

Good grief. I'm lost and confused already.

I find the simplicity of *"No thanks, I don't drink"* is much easier. You can make it a part of your identity, no further need to think about it. It's not forever, it's just 30 days. For those 30 days, you don't drink. That way, you don't have to think about it. After that, see how you feel, and decide on the next 30 days then.

At home, to yourself, your spouse, your family, whoever you live with, it's an easy message *"I'm not drinking for 30 days, for my health, I'm giving my liver a rest, you should try it too!"* Simples. Don't make a big deal out of it, play it down, *"it's just a detox"*, end of discussion.

If you have to attend any office parties, social gatherings, weddings or such like just run with *"No thanks, I'm driving"* and when they insist that you must join in with the champagne toasts, you just say *"I can't, I'm on antibiotics for a throat infection, thanks, just give me the non-alcoholic option"* and don't make a big fuss.

Keep it simple, but stand firm.

Beyond 30 days

Try the 30 days. Once you do that, you might want to keep going, to 60 days, or 90 days. You might do 30 days, then review how you feel.

It's going to be a different, personal experience, for everyone.

One person might do 30 days, then spend a year or more thinking about whether or not to try something longer. Another person might feel so much benefit by day 30 that they keep going and push right on through to a full year in the first hit, and maybe longer. I have a couple of friends who have done exactly that.

Your experience will be just that, yours.

It'll likely be different to mine, and everyone else's, and that's just the way it should be.

Never again?

Even at over eight years now, I never say *"never again"*. I just say "not right now".

    I know my all-or-nothing personality hasn't changed, and isn't likely to change any time soon. Right now, drinking again still won't sit comfortably with that personality, if I had one drink tomorrow, I know I'd be back to a bottle of wine per day within no time, probably just a few weeks or months.

    But later, maybe a couple of years from now, maybe a couple of decades from now, I'll probably enjoy a drink again. Perhaps I have goals to achieve in life first; maybe I'm still wrestling with my male ego; perhaps it's just about growing older, and wiser, and calming down. Who knows?

    I never say never, there is too much pressure on a big statement like that, it's too grandiose and final. I may drink again one day, I probably will, I may manage to become that sensible, controlled, moderate, social drinker, or I may not. I just say *"I don't drink right now."*

    And that's the whole story.

    For now, for today, that's all I need.

Your First Year

Thirty days is a great place to start. As we covered earlier, you can probably navigate your way through a 30-day period of abstinence without having to explain yourself to too many friends, relatives and colleagues if you prefer it that way.

But if you decide to push on for longer, if you are going for a 90-day challenge, or one year, or longer, then at some point, everyone is going to find out. At some point, you are going to have to deal with people questioning what you are doing and why you are doing it.

If you decide to give up alcohol completely, for a year or more, then you are going to face some changes.

The long journey

Your life will change. Importantly, your *social life* will change. Get used to that right now. I wish I had known that from the outset, it would have made my first year much easier.

One weird thing that might happen, and it's actually pretty annoying when it does, is that a handful of your friends will find it highly amusing and entertaining trying to tempt you to break your vow, give up and go back to drinking. It's annoying because you are sold on the health benefits, you've built up to this in your mind, you're trying really hard not to think about drinking, and these arseholes buy you drinks, put them under your nose, and taunt you to drink up!

Generally, the people most likely to do this will be your favourite old drinking buddies. In my experience the more you were the 'big-time party animal', the harder this will be.

I don't think these people mean to be total idiots; I don't think they realise how this is a big deal for you, and you care about this, and you are really trying hard. They just seem to think it's funny. And you can't even tell them to back off and stop trying to spoil it for you, because they just say *"See, not drinking has made you boring and moody! You're no fun!"*

Very frustrating.

Making changes

My own personal experience may not be relevant to you or to anyone else, but I'll share it anyway. For me personally, that first year off alcohol was awkward...I kept trying to still socialise in the old ways, but with me being the odd one out, the only sober one. That felt weird. The scene was familiar to me in every way - the inside of a pub, the smells, the sounds, the friends faces, only they were all drinking beer and getting drunk, and I was drinking orange juice and staying sober.

Ironically, when you tell people that you have quit drinking, one of the first things many of them say is *"Oh how boring."* There is a popular misconception that being drunk means fun, laughter, good times, and being sober means quiet, boring, sensible, serious, dull. Yet, when you are the sober person in a room full of drunk people, you soon realise how tedious they all are, and what dull, repetitive crap they all talk.

I found that first year quite hard to be honest. Me not drinking wasn't the hard bit. The hard bit was trying to socialise with my friends and tolerating them onwards from the third of fourth drink, when I was stone cold sober and they were all starting to talk utter bollocks.

In my opinion, if your social life stays the same, it's going to feel weird, probably awkward, and that's going to make it harder for you.

In time, things moved on, I found a new way:

- Not less socialising, just different socialising
- Not less interests, just different interests
- Not less fun, just different fun

Now, instead of Saturday nights with my drinking buddies, it's Sunday mornings with my running or cycling buddies. Instead of meeting friends for a few drinks and a curry, it's meeting friends for a Sunday dog walk and a nice lunch. Instead of meeting a mate in the pub for a catch up, it's in a coffee shop.

I meet friends and we go walking, cycling or running for a catch up and chat, and a coffee afterwards. Often, it's the same friends, just a change of setting. Still happy, still laughing, still good times, just that you feel better, save money, and live longer.

I have just as many friends, socialise just as often, laugh just as often, and enjoy life. The difference is I am sober, 101 pounds lighter, I don't feel like crap with a hangover the next day and I hope I'll live for an extra 20 or 30 years more. **Not boring, just different.**

Influence

Now, some years down the line, no one asks me about drinking any more. No old drinking buddies try to tempt me (well, maybe occasionally one or two still do!) No one nags, pushes, pesters, questions, or criticises. I'm old news, everyone has long forgotten about the old me, and everyone has gotten used to the new teetotal me.

Along the way, I have noticed how many friends and family have followed my lead, to one degree or another, and it's extremely reassuring to see how much positive influence I am having on other people. Some old drinking buddies, rather than laughing at me, quietly approached me and told me how inspired they felt, they were **so glad someone had stood up and made the first move**, it kinda 'gave them permission' to follow suit, they had been worried about the health impact of drinking for a long time and they were hugely grateful to have this opportunity to cut back or take a break altogether.

When dear friends say such things, it means a lot.

Go on. Lead.

Be a light in the darkness, be a beacon of hope, because you don't know who else needs it.

Go on. I dare you.

The Best Version of You

This book is an invitation to you to set yourself free of the social and cultural hypnosis of alcohol. Change your life for the better, and stop damaging your body with this legal poison.

I think people are so "lost in the fog" of life, relaxing daily by using the world's most popular 'medication', that they can't envisage a life without it. We are culturally brow-beaten into believing that drinking is cool, fun, hip and sexy, and we are told that to go without is somehow boring, and we are probably missing out on all the fun that everyone else is having.

I say clear the fog, buck the trend, be a leader, not one of the glassy-eyed sheeple, plodding along the path to dependency.

Alcohol is, in my opinion, one of the popular 'social drugs' that drain our energy, erode our health, and sedate our ambitions. It's part of something that I call 'The Triad of Self-destruction', along with refined sugar, and 'junk media' including trash TV, trash newspapers, and excessive use of social media. I believe this 'triad' of forces (alcohol, sugar, and junk media) breed apathy and drain our enthusiasm and ambition for self-improvement.

It's this apathy, this 'lost in the fog' drift through life, that drains the soul over time, rendering us spiritually numb. The years go by, we celebrate the good days with booze, we drown out the bad days with booze, and we fill the boredom in between with more booze as a distraction therapy.

I implore you to overcome apathy and get the most out of your life.
Your results are up to you.

There is no government department for mental clarity, no national mandate for personal improvement, it all comes down to you. **It's your own choice**, *no one else can shake you up and change your life for the better, it has to be you.*

You don't have to quit for life right now, don't make it too much of a big deal mentally, just decide *"I am not going to drink for* **now***"* and that may be one month, or one year, or it might be two, or three, five, even ten years or longer, who knows – you will know, what feels right to you.

Just decide to stop drinking for now, try it for the first 30 days, and then for as long as it makes you feel better, keep going.

Life is better without booze.

Make the smart choice.

Break free, be different, take control of your own destiny.

To Your Future

The aim of this short book is to get you thinking. I don't claim to be an expert on addiction therapies or any such, and while I would love to help the millions of dependent drinkers out there suffering full-blown alcoholism, I fear I am not adequately skilled to do so.

But for the millions trapped in dependency, there are **multiple millions more** who are not there *yet*, but perhaps they might be on their way, or at the very least they are drinking in a way that is *harmful to their health*, depleting their mental capacity and draining their zest and vitality.

It is my hope that you have read this book and come to see the insidious nature of alcohol, and made a decision to *participate actively* in creating a better future for yourself.

Learning

One: Face the truth: you booze, you lose. No one chooses to become an alcoholic, but we can and do choose to stack the odds in our own favour, or against us. Alcohol is an insidious poison. Know this, and make the decision to limit the power alcohol has in your life. You can help yourself. You have a choice. Choose wisely.

Two: My own story. You will recall, for me it was my *relationship* with alcohol that troubled me. I liked to drink every day, and I felt the drink had more control over me, than I had over the drink. This was an *uncomfortable realisation* for me, and it was the seed of change in my life.

Three: How 30 days became eight years. Flush with success from my first test, I wanted more. 30 days made me feel better, and 90 days more noticeably so. More energy, lost weight, clearer mind, I pushed on to one year. After one year, there was no going back, I was hooked on feeling so much better. By two years, I had mental sharpness and clearer thinking in a way I had never before experienced. The fog of life lifted, I now see the world so much clearer, in ways that before, *I never knew I was missing*.

Four: The health burden. Alcohol is a causal or contributory factor in 200 health conditions and mental health problems. Alcohol is a direct cause of seven types of cancer, liver disease, depression and various behavioural problems. The societal burden of health costs, and lost productivity caused by excessive drinking, is costing us so much it's negating GDP growth in the world's most developed nations.

Five: Your challenge. Time to stop reading about me, and get to work on *you*. Start with 30 days, come on champ, you can do 30 days. Start on a Monday, zip through the working week, make it through your first dry weekend, and once you're a week in, you've got this thing in your grasp. A new future, and a new you, is there for the taking. Go on, get cracking, I'm rooting for you.

Six: What to expect over that first year. A few friends will try to tempt you. In a word, fuck 'em. Many will think you are mad, and suggest that the new you is likely to be very boring. Ignore them. Laugh them off. Change your social life, don't make this thing harder for yourself by continuing to attend the bars, pubs, parties and drinking sessions. Keep your friends, just meet them in different social settings, where you will make more, new friends too. Don't be small. Don't be afraid. Lead, and see who follows. Trust me, in time, many will.

Seven: An invitation to be the best version of you. Booze takes the best of people, booze drains you, and breeds apathy along the way. Apathy is a killer. It kills your energy, your drive, and your ambition. It kills your dreams and steals years away from your life, ending only in mediocrity, disappointment, and regret. You have to fight that shit. Daily. Set your standards higher, raise yourself up and be the best version of yourself that you can be.

To your good health, to your sobriety, to your ongoing success.
Cheers.

One-Hour Wisdom

BECAUSE TIME IS YOUR MOST VALUABLE RESOURCE

Small Books: Big Ideas

This is the second book in the 'One-hour wisdom' series.

These books are purposefully short, not exceeding 10,000 words, designed to be read in 60 to 90 minutes, because our time is such a precious resource. There is a need to grasp important ideas, and take away something actionable, without having to wade through 500 pages to get there.

These books address that need. They deliver less reading, but not less value; please don't mistake brevity for frivolity.

Other books in this series:

Win One, Lose One, Keep Going Anyway - My first business earned me over a million in net income, then my second business struggled to take off. I had to figure out what made the difference, and I share the six lessons I learned in this book.

Available on Amazon around the world.

More

IF YOU WOULD LIKE TO GO FURTHER

Good book?

Have you enjoyed this book? Has it been useful to you?

Honest, good quality Amazon Reviews are a massive help to everyone – they help hard-working authors to reach a wider audience, and they help guide readers to good books. If you have enjoyed this book, please leave a short review on Amazon. Just a sentence or two is plenty, it would be a great help to me and it would be very much appreciated.

Thank you.

Want more?

If you are interested, check out my other books on Amazon, or check out my sites at www.KarlWhitfield.com and www.MotherNaturesDiet.com where you will find books, blogs, videos, live events and more.

You can email me at karl@mndhealth.com if you like. Please feel free to get in touch, say hi, let me know how you are getting on in your life journey, I love to hear your stories.

To your sobriety and success, cheers.

Legal Disclaimer

The information and opinions provided in this book are designed for educational purposes only, and should not be taken as a substitute for medical advice or professional care. You should always consult with your doctor if you have any concerns about your health or any specific condition, treatment or if you plan to make any change to your diet or exercise routine. Do not use the information in this document to diagnose or treat any health problems or illnesses without consulting a licenced doctor.

No warranties or representations are made as to the accuracy of the information that appears in this document or at our web sites at www.KarlWhitfield.com and www.MotherNaturesDiet.com or other sites that may be referred to in this document. If you visit websites from this document, you do so at your own risk. Any decision about your health or medical care based solely on information obtained from a commercial book, or from the Internet could be dangerous. Please consult a doctor with any questions or concerns you might have regarding your health. The author of this document cannot answer direct, personal medical queries, and cannot be held responsible for your health outcomes.

We hope that you will find information in this document of interest, but no responsibility of any nature whatsoever is accepted for any information contained in these pages. You use this information at your own risk. Karl Whitfield and MND Health Ltd are in no way liable for any use or misuse of any information obtained from this document or from our websites.

Copyright

© Karl Whitfield, MND Health Ltd. Copyright 2020

Printed in Great Britain
by Amazon